MENTAL ILLNESS AND SOCIAL POLICY

The American Experience

MENTAL ILLNESS AND SOCIAL POLICY

The American Experience

Advisory Editor
GERALD N. GROB

Editorial Board
ERIC T. CARLSON
BLANCHE D. COLL
CHARLES E. ROSENBERG

WEAR AND TEAR

OR

HINTS FOR THE OVERWORKED

BY

S. WEIR MITCHELL

ARNO PRESS
A NEW YORK TIMES COMPANY
New York • 1973

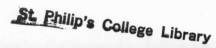

Reprint Edition 1973 by Arno Press Inc.

Reprinted from a copy in
   The College of Physicians of Philadelphia Library

MENTAL ILLNESS AND SOCIAL POLICY: ·
   The American Experience
ISBN for complete set: 0-405-05190-5
See last pages of this volume for titles.

Manufactured in the United States of America

———————◆———————

Library of Congress Cataloging in Publication Data

Mitchell, Silas Weir, 1829-1914.
   Wear and tear.

   (Mental illness and social policy: the American
experience)
   Reprint of the ed. published by Lippincott,
Philadelphia.
   1. Fatigue, Mental.   I. Title.   II. Series.
[DNLM: WM M682w 1887F]
RC351.M65 1973   614.5'823   73-2407
ISBN 0-405-05217-0

Wear and Tear,

OR

HINTS FOR THE OVERWORKED.

BY

S. WEIR MITCHELL, M.D., LL.D. Harv.,

MEMBER OF THE NATIONAL ACADEMY OF SCIENCES, PRESIDENT OF
THE COLLEGE OF PHYSICIANS OF PHILADELPHIA, ETC.

FIFTH EDITION,
THOROUGHLY REVISED.

PHILADELPHIA:
J. B. LIPPINCOTT COMPANY.
1887.

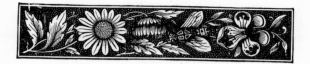

PREFACE.

THE rate of change in this country in education, in dress, and in diet and habits
of daily life surprises even the most watchful
American observer. It is now but fifteen years
since this little book was written as a warning to a restless nation possessed of an energy
tempted to its largest uses by unsurpassed op-
portunities. There is still need to repeat and
reinforce my former remonstrance, but I am
glad to add that since I first wrote on these
subjects they have not only grown into impor-
tance as questions of public hygiene, but vast
changes for the better have come about in many
of our ways of living, and everywhere common
sense is beginning to rule in matters of dress,
diet, and education.

The American of the Eastern States and

of the comfortable classes* is becoming notably more ruddy and more stout. The alteration in women as to these conditions is most striking, and, if I am not mistaken, in England there is a lessening tendency towards that excess of adipose matter which is still a surprise to the American visiting England for the first time.

I should scarcely venture to assert so positively that Americans had obviously taken on flesh within a generation if what I see had not been observed by many others. It would, I think, be interesting to enter at length upon a study of these remarkable changes, but that were scarcely within the scope of this little book.

---

* Happily, a large class with us.

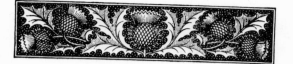

WEAR AND TEAR.

OR

HINTS FOR THE OVERWORKED.

MANY years ago* I found occasion to set before the readers of *Lippincott's Magazine* certain thoughts concerning work in America, and its results. Somewhat to my surprise, the article attracted more notice than usually falls to the share of such papers, and since then, from numerous sources, I have had the pleasure to learn that my words of warning have been of good service to many thoughtless sinners against the laws of labor and of rest. I have found, also, that the views then set forth as to the peculiar diffi-

---

* In 1871.

culties of mental and physical work in this country are in strict accordance with the personal experience of foreign scholars who have cast their lots among us; while some of our best teachers have thanked me for stating, from a doctor's stand-point, the evils which their own experience had taught them to see in our present mode of tasking the brains of the younger girls.

I hope, therefore, that I am justified in the belief that in its new and larger form my little tract may again claim attention from such as need its lessons. Since it was meant only for these, I need not excuse myself to physicians for its simplicity; while I trust that certain of my brethren may find in it enough of original thought to justify its reappearance, as its statistics were taken from manuscript notes and have been printed in no scientific journal.

I have called these, Hints WEAR and TEAR, because this title clearly and briefly points out my meaning. *Wear* is a natural and legitimate result of lawful use, and is what we all have to put up with as the result of years of activity of brain and body. *Tear* is another matter: it comes of hard or evil usage of body or engine, of putting things to wrong purposes, using a chisel for a screw-driver, a penknife for a gimlet. Long strain, or the sudden demand of strength from weakness, causes tear. Wear comes of use; tear, of abuse.

The sermon of which these words are the text has been preached many times in many ways to congregations for whom the Dollar Devil had always a more winning eloquence. Like many another man who has talked wearily to his fellows with an honest sense of what they truly need, I feel how vain it is to hope for many earnest listeners. Yet here and there may be men and women, ignorantly sinning against the laws by which they should live or should guide the lives of others, who will perhaps be willing to heed what one unbiased thinker has to say in regard to the dangers of the way they are treading with so little knowledge as to where it is leading.

The man who lives an out-door life—who sleeps with the stars visible above him—who wins his bodily subsistence at first hand from the earth and waters—is a being who defies rain and sun, has a strange sense of elastic

strength, may drink if he likes, and may
smoke all day long, and feel none the worse
for it. Some such return to the earth for the
means of life is what gives vigor and develop-
ing power to the colonist of an older race
cast on a land like ours. A few generations
of men living in such fashion store up a capital of vitality which accounts largely for the
prodigal activity displayed by their descendants,
and made possible only by the sturdy contest
with Nature which their ancestors have waged.
That such a life is still led by multitudes of
our countrymen is what alone serves to keep
up our pristine force and energy. Are we
not merely using the interest on these accu-
mulations of power, but also wastefully spending the capital? From a few we have grown
to millions, and already in many ways the
people of the Atlantic coast present the peculiarities of an old nation. Have we lived too
fast? The settlers here, as elsewhere, had
ample room, and lived sturdily by their own
hands, little troubled for the most part with
those intense competitions which make it hard
to live nowadays and embitter the daily bread
of life. Neither had they the thousand intricate

problems to solve which perplex those who struggle to-day in our teeming city hives. Above all, educational wants were limited in kind and in degree, and the physical man and woman were what the growing state most needed.

How much and what kind of good came of the gradual change in all these matters we well enough know. That in one and another way the cruel competition for the dollar, the new and exacting habits of business, the racing speed which the telegraph and railway have introduced into commercial life, the new value which great fortunes have come to possess as means towards social advancement, and the overeducation and overstraining of our young people, have brought about some great and growing evils, is what is now beginning to be distinctly felt. I should like, therefore, at the risk of being tedious, to re-examine this question—to see if it be true that the nervous system of certain classes of Americans is being sorely overtaxed—and to ascertain how much our habits, our modes of work, and, haply, climatic peculiarities, may have to do with this state of things. But before ven-

turing anew upon a subject which may pos-
sibly excite controversy and indignant comment, let me premise that I am talking chiefly
of the crowded portions of our country, of
our great towns, and especially of their upper
classes, and am dealing with those higher
questions of mental hygiene of which in general we hear but too little. If the strictures
I have to make applied as fully throughout
the land—to Oregon as to New England, to
the farmer as to the business man, to the
women of the artisan class as to those socially
above them—then indeed I should cry, God
help us and those that are to come after us!
Owing to causes which are obvious enough,
the physical worker is being better and better
paid and less and less hardly tasked, while
just the reverse obtains in increasing ratios
for those who live by the lower form of brain-
work; so that the bribe to use the hand is
growing daily, and pure mechanical labor, as
opposed to that of the clerk, is being "levelled
upward" with fortunate celerity.

Before attempting to indicate certain ways
in which we as a people are overtaxing and
misusing the organs of thought, I should be

glad to have the privilege of explaining the
terms which it is necessary to use, and of
pointing out some of the conditions under
which mental labor is performed.

The human body carries on several kinds of
manufacture, two of which—the evolution of
muscular force or motion, and intellection with
all moral activities—alone concern us here.
We are somewhat apt to antagonize these two
sets of functions, and to look upon the latter,
or brain-labor, as alone involving the use or
abuse of the nervous system. But every blow
on the anvil is as distinctly an act of the
nerve centres as are the highest mental processes. If this be so, how or why is it that
excessive muscular exertion—I mean such as
is violent and continued—does not cause the
same appalling effects as may be occasioned by
a like abuse of the nerve-organs in mental
actions of various kinds? This is not an in-
variable rule, for, as I may point out in the
way of illustration hereafter, the centres which
originate or evolve muscular power do sometimes suffer from undue taxation; but it is
certainly true that when this happens, the evil
result is rarely as severe or as lasting as when

it is the organs of mental power that have suffered.

In either form of work, physical or mental, the will acts to start the needed processes, and afterwards is chiefly regulative. In the case of bodily labor, the spinal nerve-centres are most largely called into action. Where mental or moral processes are involved, the active organs lie within the cranium. As I said just now, when we talk of an overtaxed nervous system it is usually the brain we refer to, and not the spine; and the question therefore arises, Why is it that an excess of physical labor is better borne than a like excess of mental labor? The simple answer is, that mental overwork is harder, because as a rule it is closet or counting-room or at least in-door work—sedentary, in a word. The man who is intensely using his brain is not collaterally employing any other organs, and the more intense his application the less locomotive does he become. On the other hand, however a man abuses his powers of motion in the way of work, he is at all events encouraging that collateral functional activity which mental labor discourages: he is quickening the heart, driving the blood through unused channels, hastening the breathing and increasing the secretions of the skin —all excellent results, and, even if excessive, better than a too incomplete use of these functions.

But there is more than this in the question. We do not know as yet what is the cost in expended material of mental acts as compared with motor manifestations, and here, therefore, are at fault; because, although it seems so much slighter a thing to think a little than to hit out with the power of an athlete, it may prove that the expenditure of nerve material is in the former case greater than in the latter.

When a man uses his muscles, after a time comes the feeling called fatigue—a sensation always referred to the muscles, and due most probably to the deposit in the tissues of certain substances formed during motor activity. Warned by this weariness, the man takes rest—may indeed be forced to do so; but, unless I am mistaken, he who is intensely using the brain does not feel in the common use of it any sensation referable to the organ itself which warns him that he has taxed it enough. It is apt, like a well-bred

2

creature, to get into a sort of exalted state under the stimulus of need, so that its owner feels amazed at the ease of its processes and at the sense of *wide-awakefulness* and power that accompanies them. It is only after very long misuse that the brain begins to have means of saying, "I have done enough;" and at this stage the warning comes too often in the shape of some one of the many symptoms which indicate that the organ is already talking with the tongue of disease.

I do not know how these views will be generally received, but I am sure that the personal experience of many scholars will decide them to be correct; and they serve to make clear why it is that men may not know they are abusing the organ of thought until it is already suffering deeply, and also wherefore the mind may not be as ruthlessly overworked as the legs or arms.

Whenever I have closely questioned patients or men of studious habits as to this matter, I have found that most of them, when in health, recognized no such thing as fatigue in mental action, or else I learned that what they took for this was merely that physical

senso of being tired, which arises from prolonged writing or constrained positions. The
more, I fancy, any healthy student reflects
on this matter the more clearly will he recog-
nize this fact, that very often when his brain
is at its clearest, he pauses only because his
back is weary, his eyes aching, or his fingers
tired.

This most important question, as to how a
man shall know when he has sufficiently
tasked his brain, demands a longer answer
than I can give it here; and, unfortunately,
there is no popular book since Ray's clever
and useful "Mental Hygiene," and Feuchters-
leben's "Dietetics of the Soul," both out of
print, which deals in a readable fashion with
this or kindred topics.* Many men are
warned by some sense of want of clearness
or ease in their intellectual processes. Others
are checked by a feeling of surfeit or disgust,

---

* See, now, "Brain-Work and Overwork," by H. C. Wood,
M.D.; also, "Mental Overwork and Premature Disease among
Public and Professional Men," by Ch. K. Mills, M.D.; also,
"Overwork and Sanitation in Public Schools, with Remarks
on the Production of Nervous Disease and Insanity," by Ch.
K. Mills, M.D.,—*Annals of Hygiene*, September, 1886.

which they obey or not as they are wise or
unwise. Here, for example, is in substance
the evidence of a very attentive student of his
own mental mechanism, whom we have to
thank for many charming products of his
brain. Like most scholars, he can scarcely
say that he ever has a sense of " brain-tire,"
because cold hands and feet and a certain
restlessness of the muscular system drive him
to take exercise. Especially when working at
night, he gets after a time a sense of disgust
at the work he is doing. " But sometimes,"
he adds, " my brain gets going, and is to be
stopped by none of the common plans of
counting, repeating French verbs, or the like."
A well-known poet describes to me the curious
condition of excitement into which his brain
is cast by the act of composing verse, and
thinks that the happy accomplishment of his
task is followed by a feeling of relief, which
shows that there has been high tension.

One of our ablest medical scholars reports
himself to me as having never been aware of
any sensation in the head, by which he could
tell that he had worked enough, up to a late
period of his college career, when, having

overtaxed his brain, he was restricted by his advisers to two or three hours of daily study. He thus learned to study hard, and ever since has been accustomed to execute all mental tasks at high pressure under intense strain and among the cares of a great practice. All his mind-work is, however, forced labor, and it always results in a distinct sense of cerebral fatigue,—a feeling of pressure, which is eased by clasping his hands over his head; and also there is desire to lie down and rest.

"I am not aware," writes a physician of distinction, "that, until a few years ago, I ever felt any sense of fatigue from brain-work which I could refer to the organ employed. The longer I worked the clearer and easier my mental processes seemed to be, until, during a time of great sorrow and anxiety, I pushed my thinking organs rather too hard. As a result, I began to have headache after every period of intellectual exertion. Then I lost power to sleep. Although I have partially recovered, I am now always warned when I have done enough, by lessening ease in my work, and by a sense of fulness and tension in the head." The indications of brain-tire,

b   2*

therefore, differ in different people, and are
more and more apt to be referred to the
thinking organ as it departs more and more
from a condition of health. Surely a fuller
record of the conditions under which men of
note are using their mental machinery would
be everyway worthy of attention.

Another reason why too prolonged use of
the brain is so mischievous is seen in a
peculiarity, which is of itself a proof of the
auto-activity of the vital acts of the various
organs concerned in intellection. We sternly
concentrate attention on our task, whatever it
be; we do this too long, or under circumstances which make labor difficult, such as
during digestion or when weighted by anxiety.
At last we stop and propose to find rest in
bed. Not so, says the ill-used brain, now
morbidly wide awake; and whether we will
or not, the mind keeps turning over and over
the work of the day, the business or legal
problem, or mumbling, so to speak, some
wearisome question in a fashion made useless
by the denial of full attention. Or else the
imagination soars away with the unrestful
energy of a demon, conjuring up an endless

procession of broken images and disconnected thoughts, so that sleep is utterly banished.

I have chosen here as examples men whose brains are engaged constantly in the higher forms of mental labor; but the difficulty of arresting at will the overtasked brain belongs more or less to every man who overuses this organ, and is the well-known initial symptom of numerous morbid states. I have instanced scholars and men of science chiefly, because they, more than others, are apt to study the conditions under which their thinking organs prosper or falter in their work, and because from them have we had the clearest accounts of this embarrassing condition of automatic activity of the cerebral organs. Few thinkers have failed, I fancy, to suffer in this way at some time, and with many the annoyance is only too common. I do not think the subject has received the attention it deserves, even from such thorough believers in unconscious cerebration as Maudsley. As this state of brain is fatal to sleep, and therefore to need-ful repose of brain, every sufferer has a remedy which he finds more or less available. This usually consists in some form of effort

to throw the thoughts off the track upon
which they are moving. Almost every literary
biography has some instance of this difficulty,
and some hint as to the sufferer's method of
freeing his brain from the despotism of a ruling
idea or a chain of thought.

Many years ago I heard Mr. Thackeray say
that he was sometimes haunted, when his work
was over, by the creatures he himself had sum-
moned into being, and that it was a good cor-
rective to turn over the pages of a dictionary.
Sir Walter Scott is said to have been troubled
in a similar way. A great lawyer, whom I
questioned lately as to this matter, told me
that his cure was a chapter or two of a novel,
with a cold bath before going to bed; for,
said he, quaintly, " You never take out of a
cold bath the thoughts you take into it." It
would be easy to multiply such examples.

Looking broadly at the question of the influence of excessive and prolonged use of the
brain upon the health of the nervous system,
we learn, first, that cases of cerebral exhaustion in people who live wisely are rare. Eat
regularly and exercise freely, and there is
scarce a limit to the work you may get out

of the thinking organs. But if into the life of a man whose powers are fully taxed we bring the elements of great anxiety or worry, or excessive haste, the whole machinery begins at once to work, as it were, with a dangerous amount of friction. Add to this such constant fatigue of body as some forms of business bring about, and you have all the means needed to ruin the man's power of useful labor.

I have been careful here to state that combined overwork of mind and body is doubly mischievous, because nothing is now more sure in hygienic science than that a proper alternation of physical and mental labor is best fitted to insure a lifetime of wholesome and vigorous intellectual exertion. This is probably due to several causes, but principally to the fact that during active exertion of the body the brain cannot be employed intensely, and therefore has secured to it a state of repose which even sleep is not always competent to supply. There is a Turkish proverb which occurs to me here, like most proverbs, more or less true: "Dreaming goes afoot, but who can think on horseback?" Perhaps, too,

there is concerned a physiological law, which,
though somewhat mysterious, I may again
have to summon to my aid in the way of explanation.   It is known as the law of Trevi-
ranus, its discoverer, and may thus be briefly
stated: Each organ is to every other as an
excreting organ.   In other words, to insure
perfect health, every tissue, bone, nerve,
tendon, or muscle should take from the blood
certain materials and return to it certain
others.   To do this every organ must or
ought to have its period of activity and of
rest, so as to keep the vital fluid in a proper
state to nourish every other part.   This pro-
cess in perfect health is a system of mutual
assurance, and is probably essential to a
condition of entire vigor of both mind and
body.

It has long been believed that maladies of
the nervous system are increasing rapidly in the
more crowded portions of the United States;
but I am not aware that any one has studied
the death-records to make sure of the accu-
racy of this opinion.   There can be no doubt,
I think, that the palsy of children becomes
more frequent in cities just in proportion to

their growth in population. I mention it
here because, as it is a disease which does not
kill but only cripples, it has no place in the
mortuary tables. Neuralgia is another malady
which has no record there, but is, I suspect,
increasing at a rapid rate wherever our people
are crowded together in towns. Perhaps no
other form of sickness is so sure an indication
of the development of the nervous temperament, or that condition in which there are
both feebleness and irritability of the nervous
system. But the most unquestionable proof
of the increase of nervous disease is to be
looked for in the death statistics of cities.

There, if anywhere, we shall find evidence
of the fact, because there we find in exagger-
ated shapes all the evils I have been defining.
The best mode of testing the matter is to
take the statistics of some large city which
has grown from a country town to a vast business hive within a very few years. Chicago
fulfils these conditions precisely. In 1852 it
numbered 49,407 souls. At the close of 1868
it had reached to 252,054. Within these years
it has become the keenest and most wide-
awake business centre in America. I owe to

the kindness of Dr. J. H. Rauch, Sanitary Superintendent of Chicago, manuscript records, hitherto unpublished, of its deaths from nervous disease, as well as the statement of each year's total mortality; so that I have it in my power to show the increase of deaths from nerve disorders relatively to the annual loss of life from all causes. I possess similar details as to Philadelphia, which seem to admit of the same conclusions as those drawn from the figures I have used. But here the evil has increased more slowly. Let us see what story these figures will tell us for the Western city. Unluckily, they are rather dry tale-tellers.

The honest use of the mortuary statistics of a large town is no easy matter, and I must therefore ask that I may be supposed to have taken every possible precaution in order not to exaggerate the reality of a great evil. Certain diseases, such as apoplexy, palsy, epilepsy, St. Vitus's dance, and lockjaw or tetanus, we all agree to consider as nervous maladies; convulsions, and the vast number of cases known in the death-lists as dropsy of the brain, effusion on the brain, etc., are to be looked upon with more doubt. The former, as every doctor knows, are, in a vast proportion of instances, due to direct disease of the nerve-centres; or, if not to this, then to such a condition of irritability of these parts as makes them too ready to originate spasms in response to causes which disturb the extremities of the nerves, such as teething and the like. This tendency seems to be fostered by the air and habits of great towns, and by all the agencies which in these places depress the health of a community. The other class of diseases, as dropsy of the brain or effusion, probably includes a number of maladies, due some of them to scrofula, and to the predisposing causes of that disease; others, to the kind of influences which seem to favor convulsive disorders. Less surely than the former class can these be looked upon as true nervous diseases; so that in speaking of them I am careful to make separate mention of their increase, while thinking it right on the whole to include in the general summary of this growth of nerve disorders this partially doubtful class.

Taking the years 1852 to 1868, inclusive, it will be found that the population of Chicago has increased 5.1 times and the deaths from all causes 3.7 times; while the nerve deaths, including the doubtful class labelled in the reports as dropsy of the brain and convulsions, have risen to 20.4 times what they were in 1852. Thus in 1852, '53, and '55, leaving out the cholera year '54, the deaths from nerve disorders were respectively to the whole population as 1 in 1149, 1 in 953, and 1 in 941; whilst in 1866, '67, and '68, they were 1 in 505, 1 in 415.7, and 1 in 287.8. Still omitting 1854, the average proportion of neural deaths to the total mortality was, in the five years beginning with 1852, 1 in 26.1. In the five latter years studied—that is, from 1864 to 1868, inclusive—the proportion was 1 nerve death to every 9.9 of all deaths.

I have alluded above to a class of deaths included in my tables, but containing, no doubt, instances of mortality due to other causes than disease of the nerve-organs. Thus many which are stated to have been owing to convulsions ought to be placed to the credit of tubercular disease of the brain or to heart maladies; but even in the practice of medicine the distinction as to cause cannot always be made; and as a large proportion of this loss of life is really owing to brain affections, I have thought best to include the whole class in my statement.

A glance at the individual diseases which are indubitably nervous is more instructive and less perplexing. For example, taking the extreme years, the recent increase in apoplexy is remarkable, even when we remember that it is a malady of middle and later life, and that Chicago, a new city, is therefore entitled to a yearly increasing quantity of this form of death. In 1868 the number was 8.6 times greater than in 1852. Convulsions as a death cause had in 1868 risen to 22 times as many as in the year 1852. Epilepsy, one of the most marked of all nervous maladies, is more free from the difficulties which belong to the last-mentioned class. In 1852 and '53 there were but two deaths from this disease; in the next four years there were none. From 1858 to '64, inclusive, there were in all 6 epileptic deaths: then we have in the following years, 5, 3, 11; and in 1868 the number had increased to 17. Passing over palsy, which, like apoplexy, increases in 1868,—8.6 times as compared with

1852, and 26 times as compared with the four years following 1852,—we come to lockjaw, an unmistakable nerve malady. Six years out of the first eleven give us no death from this painful disease; the others, up to 1864, offer each one only, and the last-mentioned year has but two. Then the number rises to 3 each year, to 5 in 1867, and to 12 in 1868. At first sight, this record of mortality from lockjaw would seem to be conclusive, yet it is perhaps, of all the maladies mentioned, the most deceptive as a means of determining the growth of neural diseases. To make this clear to the general reader, he need only be told that tetanus is nearly always caused by mechanical injuries, and that the natural increase of these in a place like Chicago may account for a large part of the increase. Yet, taking the record as a whole, and viewing it only with a calm desire to get at the truth, it is not possible to avoid seeing that the growth of nerve maladies has been inordinate.

The industry and energy which have built this great city on a morass, and made it a vast centre of insatiate commerce, are now at work to undermine the nervous systems of its restless and eager people,* with what result I have here tried to point out, chiefly because it is an illustration in the most concentrated form of causes which are at work elsewhere throughout the land.

The facts I have given establish the disproportionate increase in one great city of those diseases which are largely produced by the strain on the nervous system resulting from the toils and competitions of a community growing rapidly and stimulated to its utmost capacity. Probably the same rule would be found to apply to other large towns, but I have not had time to study the statistics of any of them fully; and, for reasons already given, Chicago may be taken as a typical illustration.

It were interesting to-day to question the later statistics of this great business-centre; to see if the anwers would weaken or reinforce the conclusions drawn in 1871. I have seen it anew of late with its population of 700,000 souls. It is a place to-day to excite wonder, and pity, and

---

* I asked two citizens of this uneasy town—on the same day--what was their business. Both replied tranquilly that they were speculators !

3*

fear. All the tides of its life move with bustling swiftness. Nowhere else are the streets more full, and nowhere else are the faces so expressive of preoccupation, of anxiety, of excitement. It is making money fast and accumulating a physiological debt of which that bitter creditor, the future, will one day demand payment.

If I have made myself understood, we are now prepared to apply some of our knowledge to the solution of certain awkward questions which force themselves daily upon the attention of every thoughtful and observant physician, and have thus opened a way to the discussion of the causes which, as I believe, are deeply affecting the mental and physical health of working Americans. Some of these are due to the climatic conditions under which all work must be done in this country, some are outgrowths of our modes of labor, and some go back to social habitudes and defective methods of early educational training.

In studying this subject, it will not answer to look only at the causes of sickness and weakness which affect the male sex. If the mothers of a people are sickly and weak, the sad inheritance falls upon their offspring, and this is why I must deal first, however briefly, with the health of our girls, because it is here, as the doctor well knows, that the trouble begins. Ask any physician of your acquaintance to sum up thoughtfully the young girls he knows, and to tell you how many in each score are fit to be healthy wives and mothers, or in fact to be wives and mothers at all. I have been asked this question myself very often, and I have heard it asked of others. The answers I am not going to give, chiefly because I should not be believed—a disagreeable position, in which I shall not deliberately place myself. Perhaps I ought to add that the replies I have heard given by others were appalling.

Next, I ask you to note carefully the expression and figures of the young girls whom you may chance to meet in your walks, or whom you may observe at a concert or in the ball-room. You will see many very charming faces, the like of which the world cannot match —figures somewhat too spare of flesh, and, especially south of Rhode Island, a marvellous littleness of hand and foot. But look further, and especially among New England young girls :

you will be struck with a certain hardness of line in form and feature which should not be seen between thirteen and eighteen, at least; and if you have an eye which rejoices in the tints of health, you will too often miss them on the cheeks we are now so daringly criticising. I do not want to do more than is needed of this ungracious talk: suffice it to say that multitudes of our young girls are merely pretty to look at, or not that; that their destiny is the shawl and the sofa, neuralgia, weak backs, and the varied forms of hysteria,—that domestic demon which has produced untold discomfort in many a household, and, I am almost ready to say, as much unhappiness as the husband's dram. My phrase may seem outrageously strong, but only the doctor knows what one of these self-made invalids can do to make a household wretched. Mrs. Gradgrind is, in fiction, the only successful portrait of this type of misery, of the woman who wears out and destroys generations of nursing relatives, and who, as Wendell Holmes has said, is like a vampire, sucking slowly the blood of every healthy, helpful creature within reach of her demands.

If any reader doubts my statement as to the physical failure of our city-bred women to fulfil all the natural functions of mothers, let him contrast the power of the recently imported Irish or Germans to nurse their babies a full term or longer, with that of the native women even of our mechanic classes. It is difficult to get at full statistics as to those of a higher social degree, but I suspect that not over one-half are competent to nurse their children a full year without themselves suffering gravely. I ought to add that our women, unlike ladies abroad, are usually anxious to nurse their own children, and merely cannot. The numerous artificial infant foods now for sale singularly prove the truth of this latter statement. Many physicians, with whom I have talked of this matter, believe that I do not overstate the evil; others think that two-thirds may be found reliable as nurses; while the rural doctors, who have replied to my queries, state that only from one-tenth to three-tenths of farmers' wives are unequal to this natural demand. There is indeed little doubt that the mass of our women possess that peculiar nervous organization which is associated with great

c

excitability, and, unfortunately, with less physical vigor than is to be found, for example, in
the sturdy English dames at whom Hawthorne
sneered so bitterly. And what are the causes
to which these peculiarities are to be laid?
There are many who will say that late hours,
styles of dress, prolonged dancing, etc., are to
blame; while really, with rare exceptions, the
newer fashions have been more healthy than
those they superseded, people are better clad
and better warmed than ever, and, save in
rare cases, late hours and overexertion in the
dance are utterly incapable of alone explaining
the mischief. I am far more inclined to believe that climatic peculiarities have formed
the groundwork of the evil, and enabled every
injurious agency to produce an effect which
would not in some other countries be so
severe. I am quite persuaded, indeed, that
the development of a nervous temperament
is one of the many race-changes which are
also giving us facial, vocal, and other peculiarities derived from none of our ancestral
stocks. If, as I believe, this change of temperament in a people coming largely from
the phlegmatic races is to be seen most re-

markably in the more nervous sex, it will not surprise us that it should be fostered by many causes which are fully within our own control. Given such a tendency, disease will find in it a ready prey, want of exercise will fatally increase it, and all the follies of fashion will aid in the work of ruin.

While a part of the mischief lies with climatic conditions which are utterly mysterious, the obstacles to physical exercise, arising from extremes of temperature, constitute at least one obvious cause of ill health among women in our country. The great heat of summer, and the slush and ice of winter, interfere with women who wish to take exercise, but whose arrangements to go out-of-doors involve wonderful changes of dress and an amount of preparation appalling to the masculine creature

The time taken for the more serious instruction of girls extends to the age of nineteen, and rarely over this. During some of these years they are undergoing such organic development as renders them remarkably sensitive. At seventeen I presume that healthy girls are as well able to study, *with proper precautions*, as men; but before this time overuse, or even a very steady use, of the brain is in many dangerous to health and to every probability of future womanly usefulness.

In most of our schools the hours are too many, for both girls and boys. From nine until two is, with us, the common school-time in private seminaries. The usual recess is twenty minutes or half an hour, and it is not as a rule filled by enforced exercise. In certain schools—would it were common!—ten minutes' recess is given after every hour; and in the Blind Asylum of Philadelphia this time is taken up by light gymnastics, which are obligatory. To these hours we must add the time spent in study out of school. This, for some reason, nearly always exceeds the time stated by teachers to be necessary; and most girls of our common schools and normal schools between the ages of thirteen and seventeen thus expend two or three hours. Does any physician believe that it is good for a growing girl to be so occupied seven or eight hours a day? or that it is right for her to use her brains as long a time as the mechanic employs his muscles? But this is only a part of the evil. The multiplicity of studies, the number of teachers,—each eager to get the most he can out of his pupil,—the severer drill of our day, and the greater intensity of application demanded, produce effects on the growing brain which, in a vast number of cases, can be only disastrous.

My remarks apply of course chiefly to public school life. I am glad to say that of late in all of our best school States more thought is now being given to this subject, but we have much to do before an evil which is partly a school difficulty and partly a home difficulty shall have been fully provided against.

Careful reading of our Pennsylvania reports and of those of Massachusetts convinces me that while in the country schools overwork is rare, in those of the cities it is more common, and that the system of pushing,—of competitive examinations,—of ranking, etc., is in a measure responsible for that worry which adds a dangerous element to work.

The following remarks as to the influence of home life in Massachusetts are not out of place here, and will be reinforced by what is to be said farther on by a competent authority as to Philadelphia :

4

" The danger of overwork, I believe, exists
mainly, if not wholly, in graded schools, where
large numbers are taught together, where there
is greater competition than in ungraded schools,
and where the work of each pupil cannot be
so easily adjusted to his capacity and needs.
And what are the facts in these schools? I
am prepared to agree with a recent London
School Board Report so far as to say that in
some of our graded schools there are pupils
who are overworked.   The number in any
school is, I believe, small who are stimulated
beyond their strength, and the schools are few
in which such extreme stimulation is encouraged.   When, with a large class of children
whose minds are naturally quick and active,
the teacher resorts to the daily marking of
recitations, to the giving of extra credits for
extra work done, to ranking, and to holding
up the danger of non-promotion before the
pupils; and when, added to those extra in-
ducements to work, there are given by committees and superintendents examinations for
promotion at regular intervals, it would be
very strange if there were not some pupils so
weak and so susceptible as to be encouraged

to work beyond their strength. There is another occasion of overwork which I have found in a few schools, and that is the spending of nearly all of the school time in recitation and putting off study to extra time at home. When, in a school of forty or more, pupils belong to the same class, and are not separated into divisions for recitation and study, there is a temptation to spend the greater part of the time in recitation which few teachers can resist; and if tasks are given, they have to be learned out of school or not at all. Pupils of grammar schools are known to feel obliged to study two or three hours daily from this cause at a time when they should be sleeping, or exercising in the open air. Frequently, however, it is not so much overwork as over-worry that most affects the health of the child, —that worry which may not always be traced to any fault of system or teacher, but which, it must be admitted, is too often induced by encouraging wrong motives to study.

"In making up the verdict we must not forget that others besides the teacher may be responsible for overwork and overworry. The parents and pupils themselves are quite as

often to blame as are the teachers. An un-
willingness on the part of pupils to review
work imperfectly done, and a desire on the
part of parents to have their children get into
a higher class, or to graduate, frequently cause
pupils to cram for examinations and to work
unduly at a time when the body is least able
to bear the extra strain. Again, children are
frequently required to take extra lessons in
music or some other study at home, thus de-
priving them of needed exercise and recrea-
tion, or exhausting nervous energy which is
needed for their regular school work.

"It will be observed that in this charge
against parents I do not speak of those causes
of ill health which really have nothing to do
with overwork, but which are oftentimes for-
gotten when a school-boy or girl breaks down.
I allude to the eating of improper and unwholesome food, to irregularity of eating and
sleeping, to attendance upon parties and other
places of amusement late at night, to smoking,
and to the indulgence of other habits which
tend to unduly excite the nervous system. For
very obvious reasons these causes of disease
are not brought prominently forward by the

attending physician, who doubtless thinks it safer and more flattering to his patrons to say that the child has broken down from hard study, rather than from excesses which are somewhat discreditable. While parents are clearly to blame for endangering health in the ways indicated, it may be a question whether the work required to be done in school should not be regulated accordingly; whether, in designating the studies to be taken, and in assigning lessons, there should not be taken into consideration all the circumstances of the pupil's life which can be conveniently ascertained, even though those circumstances are most unfavorable to school work and are brought about mainly through the ignorance or folly of parents. Of course there is a limit to such an adjustment of work in school, but with proper caution and a good understanding with the parents there need be little danger of advantage being taken by an indolent child; nor need the school be affected when it is understood to be a sign of weakness rather than of favor to any particular pupil to lessen his work. Not unfrequently there are found other causes of ill health than those which I have

mentioned; such, for instance, as poor ventilation, overheating of the school-room, draughts
of cold air, and the like; not to speak of the
annual public exhibition, with the possible
nervous excitement attending it. All of these
things are mentioned, not because they belong
directly to the question of overwork, but because it is well, in considering the question,
to keep in mind all possible causes of ill health,
that no one cause may be unduly emphasized." *

In private schools the same kind of thing
goes on, with the addition of foreign lan-
guages, and under the dull spur of discipline,
without the aid of any such necessities as
stimulate the pupils of what we are pleased to
call a normal (!) school.

In private schools for girls of what I may
call the leisure class of society overwork is of
course much more rare than in our normal
schools for girls, but the precocious claims of
social life and the indifference of parents as
to hours and systematic living needlessly add
to the ever-present difficulties of the school-

---

* Forty-ninth Annual Report of the Massachusetts Board
of Education, p. 204 (John T. Prince).

teacher, whose control ceases when the pupil passes out of her house.

As to the school in which both sexes are educated together a word may be said. Surely no system can be worse than that which complicates a difficult problem by taking two sets of beings of different gifts, and of unlike physiological needs and construction, and forcing them into the same educational mould.

It is a wrong for both sexes. Not much unlike the boy in childhood, there comes a time when in the rapid evolution of puberty the girl becomes for a while more than the equal of the lad, and, owing to her conscientiousness, his moral superior, but at this era of her life she is weighted by periodical disabilities which become needlessly hard to consider in a school meant to be both home and school for both sexes. Finally, there comes a time when the matured man certainly surpasses the woman in persistent energy and capacity for unbroken brain-work. If then she matches herself against him, it will be, with some exceptions, at bitter cost.

It is sad to think that the demands of civilized life are making this contest almost unavoidable. Even if we admit equality of intellect, the struggle with man is cruelly unequal and is to be avoided whenever it is possible.

The colleges for women, such as Vassar, are nowadays more careful than they were. Indeed, their machinery for guarding health while education of a high class goes on is admirable. What they still lack is a correct public feeling. The standard for health and endurance is too much that which would be normal for young men, and the sentiment of these groups of women is silently opposed to admitting that the feminine life has necessities which do not cumber that of man. Thus the unwritten code remains in a measure hostile to the accepted laws which are supposed to rule.

As concerns our colleges for young men I have little to say. The cases I see of breakdown among women between sixteen and nineteen who belong to normal schools or female colleges are out of all proportion larger than the number of like failures among young men of the same ages, and yet, as I have hinted, the arrangements for watching the health of these groups of women are usually better than such as the colleges for young men provide. The system of professional guardianship at Johns Hopkins is an admirable exception, and at some other institutions the physical examination on matriculation becomes of the utmost value, when followed up as it is in certain of these schools by compulsory physical training and occasional re-examinations of the state of health.

I do not see why the whole matter could not in all colleges be systematically made part of the examinations on entry upon studies. It would at least point out to the thoughtful student his weak points, and enable him to do his work and take his exercise with some regard to consequences. I have over and over seen young men with weak hearts or unsuspected valvular troubles who had suffered from having been allowed to play foot-ball. Cases of cerebral trouble in students, due to the use of defective eyes, are common, and I have known many valuable lives among male and female students crippled hopelessly owing to the fact that no college pre-examination of their state had taught them their true condition, and that no one had pointed out to them the necessity of such correction by glasses as would have enabled them as workers to compete on even terms with their fellows.

In a somewhat discursive fashion I have dwelt upon the mischief which is pressing to-day upon our girls of every class in life. The doctor knows how often and how earnestly he is called upon to remonstrate against this growing evil. He is, of course, well enough aware that many sturdy girls stand the strain, but he knows also that very many do not, and that the brain, sick with multiplied studies and unwholesome home life, plods on, doing poor work, until somebody wonders what is the matter with that girl; or she is left to scramble through, or break down with weak eyes, headaches, neuralgias, or what not. I am perfectly confident that I shall be told here that girls ought to be able to study hard between fourteen and eighteen years without injury, if boys can do it. Practically, how-ever, the boys of to-day are getting their toughest education later and later in life, while girls leave school at the same age as they did thirty years ago. It used to be common for boys to enter college at fourteen : at present, eighteen is a usual age of admission at Harvard or Yale. Now, let any one compare the scale of studies for both sexes employed half a century ago with that of to-day. He will find that its demands are vastly more exacting than they were,—a difference fraught with no evil for men, who attack the graver studies later in life, but most perilous for girls, who are still expected to leave school at eighteen or earlier.*

I firmly believe—and I am not alone in this opinion—that as concerns the physical future of women they would do far better if the brain were very lightly tasked and the school hours but three or four a day until they reach the age of seventeen at least. Anything, indeed, were better than loss of health; and if it be in any case a question of doubt, the school should be unhesitatingly abandoned or its hours lessened, as at least in part the source of very many of the nervous maladies with which our women are troubled. I am almost ashamed to defend a position which is held by many competent physicians, but an intelligent friend, who has read this page, still asks me why it is that overwork of brain should be so serious an

---

* Witness Richardson's heroine, who was " perfect mistress of the four rules of arithmetic"!

evil to women at the age of womanly development. My best reply would be the experience and opinions of those of us who are
called upon to see how many school-girls are
suffering in health from confinement, want of
exercise at the time of day when they most
incline to it, bad ventilation,* and too steady
occupation of mind. At no other time of life
is the nervous system so sensitive,—so irritable,
I might say,—and at no other are abundant
fresh air and exercise so important. To show
more precisely how the growing girl is injured
by the causes just mentioned would lead me to
speak of subjects unfit for full discussion in
these pages, but no thoughtful reader can be
much at a loss as to my meaning.

The following remarks I owe to the experience of a friend,† a woman, who kindly permits
me to use them in full. They complete what

---

* In the city where this is written there is, so far as I
know, not one private girls' school in a building planned
for a school-house. As a consequence, we hear endless complaints from young ladies of overheated or chilly rooms.
If the teacher be old, the room is kept too warm; if she
be young, and much afoot about her school, the apartment
is apt to be cold.

† Miss Pendleton.

I have space to add as to the matter of education, and deserve to be read with care by every parent and by every one concerned in our public schools.

" There can be no question that the health of growing girls is overtaxed; but, in my opinion, this is a vice of the age, and not primarily of the schools. I have found teachers more alive to it than parents or the general public. Upon interrogating a class of forty girls, of ages varying from twelve to fourteen, I found that more than half the number were conscious of loss of sleep and nervous apprehension before examinations; but I discovered, upon further inquiry, that nearly one-half of this class received instruction in one or two branches outside of the school curriculum, with the intention of qualifying to become teachers. I could get no information as to appetite or diet; all of the class, as the teacher informed me, being ashamed to give information on questions of the table. In the opinion of this teacher, nervousness and sleeplessness are somewhat due to studies and in-door social amusements in addition to regular school work; but chiefly to ignorance in the home as to the simplest

c   d   5

rules of healthy living. Nearly all the girls in this class drink a cup of tea before leaving home, eat a sweet biscuit as they walk, hurried and late, to school, and nothing else until they go home to their dinners at two o'clock. All their brain-work in the school-room is done before eating any nourishing food. The teacher realized the injurious effects of the present forcing system, and suggested withdrawing the girls from school for one year between the grammar- and high-school grades. When I asked whether a better result would not be obtained by keeping the girls in school during this additional year, but relieving the pressure of purely mental work by the introduction throughout all the grades of branches in household economy, she said this seemed to her ideal, but, she feared, impracticable, not from the nature of schools, but from the nature of boards.

"A Latin graduating class of seven girls, aged seventeen and eighteen years, stated that they do their work without nervousness, restlessness, or apprehension.

"This, with other statistics, would seem to bear out your theory that after seventeen girls may study with much less risk to health.

" So far as I have observed, the strain or tear is chiefly in the case of girls studying to become teachers. These girls often press forward too rapidly for the purpose of becoming self-supporting at the age of eighteen. The bait of a salary, and a good salary for one entering upon a profession, lures them on; and a false sympathy in members of boards and committees lends itself to this injurious cramming.

" Our own normal school,* which is doing a great, an indispensable, work in preparing a trained body of faithful, intelligent teachers, has succumbed to this injurious tendency. We have here the high and normal grades merged into one, the period of adolescence stricken out of the girl's school life, and many hundreds of girls hurried annually forward beyond their physical or mental capacity, in advance of their physical growth, for the sake of those who cannot afford to remain in school one or two years longer. I say this notwithstanding the fact that this school is, in my opinion, one of the most potent agencies for good in the community.

---

* Philadelphia.

" Overpressure in school appears to me to be a disease of the body politic from which this member suffers; but it also seems to me that this vast school system is the most powerful agency for the correction of the evil. In the case of girls, the first principle to be recognized is that the education of women is a problem by itself; that, in all its lower grades at all events, it is not to be laid down exactly upon the lines of education for boys.

" The school system may be made a forceful agency for building up the family, and the integrity of the home is without doubt the vital question of the age.

" Edward Everett Hale, with his far spiritual sight, has discerned the necessity for restoring home training, and advocates, to this end, short school terms of a few weeks annually. It is probable that in the future many school departments will be relegated to the home, but the homes are not now prepared to assume these duties.

" When it was discovered that citizens must be prepared for their political duties the schools were opened; but the means so far became an end that even women were educated only in the directions which bear upon public and not upon household economy. The words of Stein, that 'what we put into the schools will come out in the manhood of the nation afterward,' cannot be too often quoted. Let branches in household economy be connected with all the general as distinguished from normal-school grades, and we not only relieve the girl immediately of the strain of working with insufficient food, and of acquiring skill in household duties in addition to the school curriculum, we not only simplify and harmonize her work, but we send out in every case a woman prepared to carry this new influence into all her future life, even if a large number of these women should eventually pursue special or higher technical branches; for we are women before we are teachers, lawyers, physicians, etc., and if we are to add anything of distinctive value to the world by entering upon the fields of work hitherto pre-empted by men, it will be by the essential quality of this new feminine element.

"The strain in all work comes chiefly from lack of qualification by training or nature for the work in hand,—tear in place of wear. The schools can restore the ideal of quiet work. They have an immense advantage in regularity, discipline, time. This vast system gives an opportunity, such as no private schools offer, for ascertaining the average work which is healthful for growing girls. It is quite possible to ascertain, whether by women medical officers appointed to this end, or by the teachers themselves, the physical capacity of each girl, and to place her where this will not be exceeded. Girls trained in school under such wise supervision would go out into life qualified to guard the children of the future. The chief cause of overwork of children at present is the ignorance of parents as to the injurious effects of overwork, and of the signs of its influence.

" The first step toward the relief of overpressure and false stimulus is to discard the pernicious idea that it is the function of the normal school to offer to every girl in the community the opportunity for becoming a teacher. This unwholesome feature is the one distinctive strain which must be removed from the system. It can be done provided public and political sentiment approve. The normal school should be only a device for securing the best possible body of teachers. It should be technical.

"Every teacher knows that the average girl of seventeen has not reached the physical, mental, or moral development necessary to enter upon this severe and high professional course of studies, and that one year is insufficient for such a course.

"Lengthen the time given to normal instruction,—make it two years; give in this school instruction purely in the science of education; relegate all general instruction to a good high school covering a term of four years. In this as in all other progressive formative periods the way out is ahead.

"It will be time enough to talk of doing away with a portion of the girls' school year when the schools have fulfilled their high mission, when they have sent out a large body of American women prepared, not for a single profession, even the high feminine vocation of pedagogy, but equipped for her highest, most general and congenial functions as the source and centre of the home."

I am unwilling to leave this subject without

a few words as to our remedy, especially as concerns our public schools and normal schools for girls. What seems to me to be needed most is what the woman would bring into our school boards. Surely it is also possible for female teachers to talk frankly to that class of girls who learn little of the demands of health from uneducated or busy or careless mothers, and it would be as easy, if school boards were what they should be, to insist on such instruction, and to make sure that the claims of maturing womanhood are considered and attended to. Should I be told that this is impracticable, I reply that as high an authority as Samuel Eliot, of Massachusetts, has shown in large schools that it is both possible and valuable. As concerns the home life, it is also easy to get at the parents by annual circulars enforcing good counsel as to some of the simplest hygienic needs in the way of sleep, hours of study, light, and meals.

It were better not to educate girls at all between the ages of fourteen and eighteen, unless it can be done with careful reference to their bodily health. To-day, the American woman is, to speak plainly, too often physically unfit for her duties as woman, and is perhaps of all civilized females the least qualified to undertake those weightier tasks which tax so heavily the nervous system of man. She is not fairly up to what nature asks from her as wife and mother. How will she sustain herself under the pressure of those yet more exacting duties which nowadays she is eager to share with the man?

While making these stringent criticisms, I am anxious not to be misunderstood. The point which above all others I wish to make is this, that owing chiefly to peculiarities of climate, our growing girls are endowed with organizations so highly sensitive and impressionable that we expose them to needless dangers when we attempt to overtax them mentally. In any country the effects of such a course must be evil, but in America I believe it to be most disastrous.

As I have spoken of climate in the broad sense as accountable for some peculiarities of the health of our women, so also would I admit it as one of the chief reasons why work among men results so frequently in tear as well as wear. I believe that something in

our country makes intellectual work of all
kinds harder to do than it is in Europe; and
since we do it with a terrible energy, the
result shows in wear very soon, and almost
always in the way of tear also. Perhaps few
persons who look for evidence of this fact at
our national career alone will be willing to
admit my proposition, but among the higher
intellectual workers, such as astronomers, physi-
cists, and naturalists, I have frequently heard
this belief expressed, and by none so positively
as those who have lived on both continents.
Since this paper was first written I have been
at some pains to learn directly from Europeans
who have come to reside in America how this
question has been answered by their experience.
For obvious reasons, I do not name my wit-
nesses, who are numerous; but, although they
vary somewhat in the proportion of the effects
which they ascribe to climate and to such
domestic peculiarities as the overheating of our
houses, they are at one as regards the simple
fact that, for some reason, mental work is more
exhausting here than in Europe; while, as a
rule, such Americans as have worked abroad
are well aware that in France and in England

intellectual labor is less trying than it is with us. A great physiologist, well known among us, long ago expressed to me the same opinion; and one of the greatest of living naturalists, who is honored alike on both continents, is positive that brain-work is harder and more hurtful here than abroad,—an opinion which is shared by Oliver Wendell Holmes and other competent observers. Certain it is that our thinkers of the classes named are apt to break down with what the doctor knows as cerebral exhaustion,—a condition in which the mental organs become more or less completely incapacitated for labor,—and that this state of things is very much less common among the savans of Europe. A share in the production of this evil may perhaps be due to certain general habits of life which fall with equal weight of mischief upon many classes of busy men, as I shall presently point out. Still, these will not altogether account for the fact, nor is it to my mind explained by any of the more obvious faults in our climate, nor yet by our habits of life, such as furnace-warmed houses, hasty meals, bad cooking, or neglect of exercise. Let a man live as he may, I believe he will still discover that mental labor is with us more exhausting than we could wish it to be. Why this is I cannot say, but it is not more mysterious than the fact that agents which, as sedatives or excitants, affect the great nerve-centres, do this very differently in different climates. There is some evidence to show that this is also the case with narcotics; and perhaps a partial explanation may be found in the manner in which the excretions are controlled by external temperatures, as well as by the fact which Dr. Brown-Séquard discovered, and which I have frequently corroborated, that many poisons are retarded in their action by placing the animal affected in a warm atmosphere.

It is possible to drink with safety in England quantities of wine which here would be disagreeable in their first effect and perilous in their ultimate results. The Cuban who takes coffee enormously at home, and smokes endlessly, can do here neither the one nor the other to the same degree. And so also the amount of excitation from work which the brain will bear varies exceedingly with variations of climatic influences.

We are all of us familiar with the fact that physical work is more or less exhausting in different climates, and as I am dealing, or about to deal, with the work of business men, which involves a certain share of corporal exertion, as well as with that of mere scholars, I must ask leave to digress, in order to show that in this part of the country at least the work of the body probably occasions more strain than in Europe, and is followed by greater sense of fatigue.

The question is certainly a large one, and should include a consideration of matters connected with food and stimulants, on which I can but touch. I have carefully questioned a number of master-mechanics who employ both foreigners and native Americans, and I am assured that the British workman finds labor more trying here than at home; while perhaps the eight-hour movement may be looked upon as an instinctive expression of the main fact as regards our working class in general.

A distinguished English scholar informs me that since he has resided among us the same complaints, as to the depressing effects of physical labor in America, have come to him from

6

skilled English mechanics. What share change
of diet and the like may have in the matter I
have not space to discuss.*

Although, from what I have seen, I should
judge that overtasked men of science are especially liable to the trouble which I have
called cerebral exhaustion, all classes of men
who use the brain severely, and who have also
—and this is important—seasons of excessive
anxiety or of grave responsiblity, are subject
to the same form of disease; and this I presume is why we meet with numerous instances
of nervous exhaustion among merchants and
manufacturers. The lawyer and clergyman
offer examples, but I do not remember to have
seen many bad cases among physicians. Dis-
missing the easy jest which the latter state-

---

* The new emigrant suffers in a high degree from the
same evils as to cookery which affect only less severely the
mass of our people, and this, no doubt, helps to enfeeble
him. The frying-pan has, I fear, a better right to be called
our national emblem than the eagle, and I grieve to say it
reigns supreme west of the Alleghanies. I well remember
that a party of friends about to camp out were unable to
buy a gridiron in two Western towns, each numbering over
four thousand eaters of fried meats.

ment will surely suggest, the reason for this we may presently encounter.

My note-books seem to show that manufacturers and certain classes of railway officials are the most liable to suffer from neural exhaustion. Next to these come merchants in general, brokers, etc.; then less frequently clergymen; still less often lawyers; and more rarely doctors; while distressing cases are apt to occur among the overschooled young of both sexes.

The worst instances to be met with are among young men suddenly cast into business positions involving weighty responsibility. I can recall several cases of men under or just over twenty-one who have lost health while attempting to carry the responsibilities of great manufactories. Excited and stimulated by the pride of such a charge, they have worked with a certain exaltation of brain, and, achieving success, have been stricken down in the moment of triumph. This too frequent practice of immature men going into business, especially with borrowed capital, is a serious evil. The same person, gradually trained to naturally and slowly increasing burdens, would have been

sure of healthy success. In individual cases
I have found it so often vain to remonstrate
or to point out the various habits which col-
lectively act for mischief on our business class
that I may well despair of doing good by a
mere general statement. As I have noted
them, connected with cases of overwork, they
are these: late hours of work, irregular meals
bolted in haste away from home, the want of
holidays and of pursuits outside of business, and
the consequent practice of carrying home, as
the only subject of talk, the cares and successes
of the counting-house and the stock-board.
Most of these evil habits require no comment.
What, indeed, can be said? The man who has
worked hard all day, and lunched or dined
hastily, comes home or goes to the club to con-
verse—save the mark!—about goods and stocks.
Holidays, except in summer, he knows not,
and it is then thought time enough taken from
work if the man sleeps in the country and
comes into a hot city daily, or at the best has
a week or two at the sea-shore. This incessant monotony tells in the end. Men have
confessed to me that for twenty years they had
worked every day, often travelling at night or

on Sundays to save time, and that in all this period they had not taken one day for play. These are extreme instances, but they are also in a measure representative of a frightfully general social evil.

Is it any wonder if asylums for the insane gape for such men? There comes to them at last a season of business embarrassment; or, when they get to be fifty or thereabouts, the brain begins to feel the strain, and just as they are thinking, "Now we will stop and enjoy ourselves," the brain, which, slave-like, never murmurs until it breaks out into open insurrection, suddenly refuses to work, and the mischief is done. There are therefore two periods of existence especially prone to those troubles, —one when the mind is maturing; another at the turning-point of life, when the brain has attained its fullest power, and has left behind it accomplished the larger part of its best enterprise and most active labor.

I am disposed to think that the variety of work done by lawyers, their long summer holiday, their more general cultivation, their usual tastes for literary or other objects out of their business walks, may, to some extent,

6*

save them, as well as the fact that they can
rarely be subject to the sudden and fearful responsibilities of business men. Moreover, like
the doctor, the lawyer gets his weight upon
him slowly, and is thirty at least before it can
be heavy enough to task him severely. The
business man's only limitation is need of
money, and few young mercantile men will
hesitate to enter trade on their own account if
they can command capital. With the doctor, as
with the lawyer, a long intellectual education, a
slowly-increasing strain, and responsibilities of
gradual growth tend, with his out-door life, to
save him from the form of disease I have been
alluding to. This element of open-air life, I suspect, has a share in protecting men who in many
respects lead a most unhealthy existence. The
doctor, who is supposed to get a large share of
exercise, in reality gets very little after he grows
too busy to walk, and has then only the inci-
dental exposure to out-of-door air. When this
is associated with a fair share of physical exertion, it is an immense safeguard against the
ills of anxiety and too much brain-work. For
these reasons I do not doubt that the effects of
our great civil war were far more severely felt

by the Secretary of War and President Lincoln than by Grant or Sherman.

The wearing, incessant cares of overwork, of business anxiety, and the like, produce directly diseases of the nervous system, and are also the fertile parents of dyspepsia, consumption, and maladies of the heart. How often we can trace all the forms of the first-named protean disease to such causes is only too well known to every physician, and their connection with cardiac troubles is also well understood. Happily, functional troubles of heart or stomach are far from unfrequent precursors of the graver mischief which finally falls upon the nerve-centres if the lighter warnings have been neglected; and for this reason no man who has to use his brain energetically and for long periods can afford to disregard the hints which he gets from attacks of palpitation of heart or from a disordered stomach. In many instances these are the only expressions of the fact that he is abusing the machinery of mind or body; and the sufferer may think himself fortunate that this is the case, since even the least serious degrees of direct exhaustion of the centres with which he feels and thinks are more grave and are less open to ready relief.

When affections of the outlying organs are neglected, and even in many cases where these have not suffered at all, we are apt to witness, as a result of too prolonged anxiety combined with business cares, or even of mere overwork alone, with want of proper physical habits as to exercise, amusement, and diet, that form of disorder of which I have already spoken as cerebral exhaustion; and before closing this paper I am tempted to describe briefly the symptoms which warn of its approach or tell of its complete possession of the unhappy victim. Why it should be so difficult of relief is hard to comprehend, until we remember that the brain is apt to go on doing its weary work automatically and despite the will of the unlucky owner; so that it gets no thorough rest, and is in the hapless position of a broken limb which is expected to knit while still in use. Where physical overwork has worn out the spinal or motor centres, it is, on the other hand, easy to enforce repose, and so to place them in the best condition for repair. This was often and happily illustrated during the

late war. Severe marches, bad food, and other
causes which make war exhausting, were constantly in action, until certain men were doing
their work with too small a margin of reserve-
power. Then came such a crisis as the last
days of McClellan's retreat to the James River,
or the forced march of the Sixth Army Corps
to Gettysburg, and at once these men succumbed with palsy of the legs   A few months
of absolute rest, good diet, ale, fresh beef and
vegetables restored them to perfect health.

In all probability incessant use of a part
flushes with blood the nerve-centres which
furnish it with motor energy, so that excessive work may bring about a state of conges-
tion, owing to which the nerve-centre becomes
badly nourished, and at last strikes work. In
civil life we sometimes meet with such cases
among certain classes of artisans: paralysis of
the legs as a result of using the treadle of the
sewing-machine ten hours a day is a good example, and, I am sorry to add, not a very rare
one, among the overtasked women who slave
at such labor.

Now let us see what happens when the intellectual organs are put over-long on the

stretch, and when moral causes, such as heavy responsibilities and over-anxiety, are at work.

When in active use, the thinking organs become full of blood, and, as has been shown, rise in temperature, while the feet and hands become cold. Nature meant that, for their work, they should be, in the first place, supplied with food; next, that they should have certain intervals of rest to rid themselves of the excess of blood accumulated during their periods of activity, and this is to be done by sleep, and also by bringing into play the physical machinery of the body, such as the muscles,—that is to say, by exercise which flushes the parts engaged in it and so depletes the brain. She meant, also, that the various brain-organs should aid in the relief, by being used in other directions than mere thought; and lastly, she desired that, during digestion, all the surplus blood of the body should go to the stomach, intestines, and liver, and that neither blood nor nerve-power should be then misdirected upon the brain: in other words, she did not mean that we should try to carry on, with equal energy, two kinds of important functional business at once.

If, then, the brain-user wishes to be healthy,

he must limit his hours of work according to rules which will come of experience, and which no man can lay down for him. Above all, let him eat regularly and not at too long intervals. I well remember the amazement of a distinguished naturalist when told that his sleeplessness and irregular pulse were due to his fasting from nine until six. A biscuit and a glass of porter, at one o'clock, effected a ready and pleasant cure. As to exercise in the fresh air, I need say little, except that if the exercise can be made to have a distinct object, not in the way of business, so much the better. Nor should I need to add that we may relieve the thinking and worrying mechanisms by light reading and other amusements, or enforce the lesson that no hard work should be attempted during digestion. The wise doctor may haply smile at the commonplace of such directions, but woe be to the man who neglects them!

When an overworked and worried victim has sufficiently sinned against these simple laws, if he does not luckily suffer from disturbances of heart or stomach, he begins to have certain signs of nervous exhaustion.

As a rule, one of two symptoms appears

first, though sometimes both come together. Work gets to be a little less facile; this astonishes the subject, especially if he has been under high pressure and doing his tasks with that ease which comes of excitement. With this, or a little later, he discovers that he sleeps badly, and that the thoughts of the day infest his dreams, or so possess him as to make slumber difficult. Unrefreshed, he rises and plunges anew into the labor for which he is no longer competent. Let him stop here; he has had his warning. Day after day the work grows more trying, but the varied stimulants to exertion come into play, the mind, aroused, forgets in the cares of the day the weariness of the night season, and so, with lessening power and growing burden, he pursues his purpose. At last come certain new symptoms, such as giddiness, dimness of sight, neuralgia of the face or scalp, with entire nights of insomnia and growing difficulty in the use of the mental powers; so that to attempt a calculation, or any form of intellectual labor, is to insure a sense of distress in the head, or such absolute pain as proves how deeply the organs concerned have suffered.

Even to read is sometimes almost impossible;
and there still remains the perilous fact that
under enough of moral stimulus the man may
be able, for a few hours, to plunge into business cares, without such pain as completely to
incapacitate him for immediate activity. Night,
however, never fails to bring the punishment;
and at last the slightest prolonged exertion of
mind becomes impossible. In the worst cases
the scalp itself grows sore, and a sudden jar
hurts the brain, or seems to do so, while the
mere act of stepping from a curb-stone pro-
duces positive pain.

Strange as it may seem, much of all this
may happen to a man, and he may still struggle onward, ignorant of the terrible demands he
is making upon an exhausted brain. Usually,
by this time he has sought advice, and, if his
doctor be worthy of the title, has learned that
while there are certain aids for his symptoms
in the shape of drugs, there is only one real
remedy. Happy he if not too late in discover-
ing that complete and prolonged cessation from
work is the one thing needful. Not a week of
holiday, or a month, but probably a year or
more of utter idleness may be absolutely essen-

tial.   Only this will answer in cases so extreme
as that which I have tried to depict, and even
this will not always insure a return to a state
of active working health.

I am very far from conceding that the vehe-
ment energy with which we do our work is
due altogether to greed.   We probably idle
less and play less than any other race, and the
absence of national habits of sport, especially
in the West, leaves the man of business with
no inducement to abandon that unceasing labor
in which at last he finds his sole pleasure.   He
does not ride, or shoot, or fish, or play any
game but euchre.   Business absorbs him utterly,
and at last he finds neither time nor desire for
books.   The newspaper is his sole literature;
he has never had time to acquire a taste for
any reading save his ledger.   Honest friendship
for books comes with youth or, as a rule, not
at all.   At last his hour of peril arrives.   Then
you may separate him from business, but you
will find that to divorce his thoughts from it
is impossible.   The fiend of work he raised no
man can lay.   As to foreign travel, it wearies
him.   He has not the culture which makes
it available or pleasant.   Notwithstanding the

plasticity of the American, he is now without resources. What then to advise I have asked myself countless times. Let him at least look to it that his boys go not the same evil road. The best business men are apt to think that their own successful careers represent the lives their children ought to follow, and that the four years of college spoil a lad for business. In reality these years, be they idle or well filled with work, give young men the custom of play, and surround them with an atmosphere of culture which leaves them with bountiful resources for hours of leisure, while they insure to them in these years of growth wholesome, unworried freedom from such business pressure as the successful parent is so apt to put on too youthful shoulders.

Somewhat distracted by the desire to be brief, and yet to tell the whole story, I have sought, in what I fear is a very loose and disconnected way, to put in a new light some of the evils which are hurting the mothers of our race, and those which every day's experience teaches the doctor are gravely affecting the working capacity of numberless men. I trust I have succeeded in satisfying my readers that we dwell in a climate where work of all kinds demands greater precautions as to health than is the case abroad. We cannot improve our climate, but it is quite possible that we have not sufficiently learned to modify the conditions of labor in accordance with those of the sky under which we live.

No student of the nervous maladies of American men and women will think I have overdrawn any part of the foregoing sketch. It would have been as easy, had such a course been proper, to tell the individual stories of youth, vigorous, eager, making haste to be rich, wrecked and made unproductive and dependent for years or forever; and of middle age, unable or unwilling to pause in the career of dollar-getting, crushed to earth in the hour of fruition, or made powerless to labor longer at any cost for those who were dearest.

THE END.

MENTAL ILLNESS AND SOCIAL POLICY
THE AMERICAN EXPERIENCE

AN ARNO PRESS COLLECTION

Barr, Martin W. Mental Defectives: Their History, Treatment and Training. 1904.

The Beginnings of American Psychiatric Thought and Practice: Five Accounts, 1811-1830. 1973

The Beginnings of Mental Hygiene in America: Three Selected Essays, 1833-1850. 1973

Briggs, L. Vernon, et al. History of the Psychopathic Hospital, Boston, Massachusetts. 1922

Briggs, L. Vernon. Occupation as a Substitute for Restraint in the Treatment of the Mentally Ill. 1923

Brigham, Amariah. An Inquiry Concerning the Diseases and Functions of the Brain, the Spinal Cord, and the Nerves. 1840

Brigham, Amariah. Observations on the Influence of Religion upon the Health and Physical Welfare of Mankind. 1835

Brill, A. A. Fundamental Conceptions of Psychoanalysis. 1921

Bucknill, John Charles. Notes on Asylums for the Insane in America. 1876

Conolly, John. The Treatment of the Insane Without Mechanical Restraints. 1856

Coriat, Isador H. What is Psychoanalysis? 1917

Deutsch, Albert. The Shame of the States. 1948

Dewey, Richard. Recollections of Richard Dewey: Pioneer in American Psychiatry. 1936

Earle, Pliny. Memoirs of Pliny Earle, M. D. with Extracts from his Diary and Letters (1830-1892) and Selections from his Professional Writings (1839-1891). 1898

Galt, John M. The Treatment of Insanity. 1846

Goddard, Henry Herbert. Feeble-mindedness: Its Causes and Consequences. 1926

Hammond, William A. A Treatise on Insanity in Its Medical Relations. 1883

Hazard, Thomas R. Report on the Poor and Insane in Rhode-Island. 1851

Hurd, Henry M., editor. The Institutional Care of the Insane in the United States and Canada. 1916/1917. Four volumes.

Kirkbride, Thomas S. On the Construction, Organization, and General Arrangements of Hospitals for the Insane. 1880

Meyer, Adolf. The Commonsense Psychiatry of Dr. Adolf Meyer: Fifty-two Selected Papers. 1948

Mitchell, S. Weir. Wear and Tear, or Hints for the Overworked. 1887

Morton, Thomas G. The History of the Pennsylvania Hospital, 1751-1895. 1895

Ordronaux, John. Jurisprudence in Medicine in Relation to the Law. 1869

The Origins of the State Mental Hospital in America: Six Documentary Studies, 1837-1856. 1973

Packard, Mrs. E. P. W. Modern Persecution, or Insane Asylums Unveiled, As Demonstrated by the Report of the Investigating Committee of the Legislature of Illinois. 1875. Two volumes in one

Prichard, James C. A Treatise on Insanity and Other Disorders Affecting the Mind. 1837

Prince, Morton. The Unconscious: The Fundamentals of Human Personality Normal and Abnormal. 1921

Putnam, James Jackson. Human Motives. 1915

Russell, William Logie. The New York Hospital: A History of the Psychiatric Service, 1771-1936. 1945

Sidis, Boris. The Psychology of Suggestion: A Research into the Subconscious Nature of Man and Society. 1899

Southard, Elmer E. Shell-Shock and Other Neuropsychiatric Problems Presented in Five Hundred and Eighty-Nine Case Histories from the War Literature, 1914-1918. 1919

Southard, E[lmer] E. and Mary C. Jarrett. The Kingdom of Evils. 1922

Southard, E[lmer] E. and H[arry] C. Solomon. Neurosyphilis: Modern Systematic Diagnosis and Treatment Presented in One Hundred and Thirty-seven Case Histories. 1917

Spitzka, E[dward] C. Insanity: Its Classification, Diagnosis and Treatment. 1887

Supreme Court Holding a Criminal Term, No. 14056. The United States vs. Charles J. Guiteau. 1881/1882. Two volumes

Trezevant, Daniel H. Letters to his Excellency Governor Manning on the Lunatic Asylum. 1854

Tuke, D[aniel] Hack. The Insane in the United States and Canada. 1885

Upham, Thomas C. Outlines of Imperfect and Disordered Mental Action. 1868

White, William A[lanson]. Twentieth Century Psychiatry: Its Contribution to Man's Knowledge of Himself. 1936

Willard, Sylvester D. Report on the Condition of the Insane Poor in the County Poor Houses of New York. 1865